DIABETES IN SOUTH ASIAN PEOPLE EXPLAINED

DIABETES IN SOUTH ASIAN PEOPLE EXPLAINED

Tahseen A. Chowdhury MD FRCP
Consultant in Diabetes, Barts and the London NHS Trust,
Department of Diabetes and Metabolism, The Royal London Hospital,
London

Laila T. King RGN DSN BA MA
Warwick Medical School Education Facilitator, University of Warwick,
Coventry

ALTMAN

Published by Altman Publishing, 7 Ash Copse, Bricket Wood, St Albans, Herts, AL2 3YA

First edition 2007

Typeset in 10/12.5 Optima by Phoenix Photosetting, Chatham, Kent
Printed in Great Britain by Chiltern Printers (Slough) Ltd

ISBN 13: 978-1-86036-038-1

∞ Printed on acid-free text paper, manufactured in accordance with ANSI/NISO Z39.48-1992 (Permanence of Paper)

CONTENTS

ABOUT THE AUTHORS

Tahseen Chowdhury is Lead Clinician in Diabetes and Metabolism at the Royal London Hospital, London, and Honorary Senior Lecturer at Queen Mary University of London. His principal clinical and research interests are in management of diabetes in South Asians, diabetes and related kidney problems, and in the prevention of diabetes in South Asians. He runs a large diabetes service in East London, where over 50% of his patients are of Bangladeshi origin. He is involved in a number of clinical trials of innovative treatments for diabetes and its complications, and has published widely in peer-reviewed publications on a variety of diabetes-related topics.

Laila King was born in Finland and came to the UK to complete her PhD studies in Linguistics at Reading University. However, she moved into nursing after a period of personal illness and progressed in her career from acute medicine, CCU, palliative care, through general and specialist surgery, finally to diabetes. The incentive for the last move was her youngest daughter, Arabella, developing type 1 diabetes at the age of 5. During the past decade, Laila has worked as Diabetes Specialist Nurse in both primary and secondary care. Her passion has always been seeing the condition from the patient's point of view. As the Diabetes Specialist Educator in Tower Hamlets, she has been responsible for setting up and facilitating structured group education for patients and their carers as well as clinical education for health care professionals. Laila has developed a CD of Diabetes Information Leaflets for local use. Among her written publications are diabetes-related articles 'Impaired Wound Healing in Diabetes' and 'Insulin Injection Technique'. Recently, she has been appointed to the post of Diabetes Education Facilitator at Warwick University Medical School.

PREFACE

This book is aimed at people of South Asian origin – people who originate from Bangladesh, India, Pakistan and Sri Lanka.

Most South Asian people will know someone who has diabetes. This is because one in three South Asian people will develop diabetes during their lifetime. The condition is common, and becoming more common, not only in developed countries, but also in countries at the forefront of economic change – India and China. By 2030, it is predicted that over one-third of all people with diabetes will be from the Indian subcontinent.

You may have bought, or been given this book for a number of reasons. You may have recently been diagnosed with diabetes, or have a relative or spouse with the condition. You may have been told you are at risk of developing diabetes, or have 'borderline diabetes'. Alternatively, you may be just curious to know more about the condition, and how it can affect people. We hope that this book will help explain, in simple terms, what the diagnosis means, how it can affect those who have it, how you can reduce the risk of complications, and most importantly, how you can live a long, fulfilling and happy life with this condition.

1   WHAT IS DIABETES MELLITUS?

How was diabetes named?

Diabetes mellitus was first described in the second century AD by a Greek physician called Areteus. The word 'diabetes' comes from the Greek word for 'siphon', in the sense of 'passing through', and the word 'mellitus' which also has a Greek origin meaning 'honey' or 'sweet'. Taken together, the term implies sweetness passing through the body, and one of the main symptoms of the condition is sugar in the urine. An early test for diabetes was for the doctor to taste the urine to see if it was sweet. (Note: diabetes mellitus must be distinguished from the rarer and unrelated condition called 'diabetes insipidus', which has nothing to do with sugar, and in which patients pass a large amount of dilute urine).

What happens to sugar (glucose) in our bodies?

Diabetes is a condition characterised by high levels of **glucose** (sugar) in the blood. Glucose is the main fuel for our bodies, and is necessary to help us have energy to live, eat, breathe and move. Glucose is found in many foods, including fruit, bread and staples such as rice and potatoes (see dietary advice later). When foods containing glucose are eaten, they are broken down in the stomach and small intestine, and absorbed into the bloodstream. Once in the bloodstream, glucose needs to get into the cells where it is needed. All cells of the body require glucose, but the most important areas where glucose is taken up are:

- muscles: to help our heart to beat, and our bodies to move
- liver: to process glucose and store excess glucose for later use
- fat tissue: to convert glucose into fat for storage for future use.

There is a substance (known as a hormone) in our bloodstream that enables glucose to go into the cells of our body. This hormone is called **insulin**. Insulin is made and released by the **pancreas**, which is located in the middle of the abdomen behind the stomach. The pancreas has two

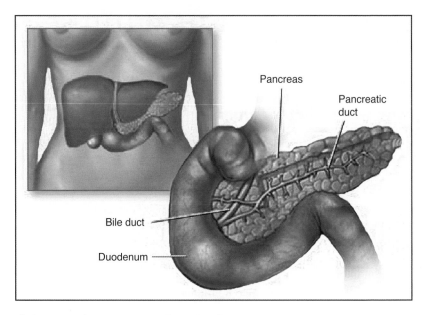

Figure 1.1 The pancreas produces insulin.

separate roles: it produces enzymes to help us break down food in the stomach and small intestine, and it also produces insulin into the bloodstream, in response to rising glucose levels. The cells in the pancreas that produce insulin are called **pancreatic beta cells**. Once released into the blood, insulin attaches to cells in the body, and opens up channels to enable glucose to enter the cells, to be used for the production of energy.

What goes wrong in diabetes?

In diabetes, there are usually two problems:

- Insulin resistance. For some reason (as yet unknown), the body does not respond to insulin as it should, and much greater levels of insulin are required to allow the glucose to enter the cells. We do not know why this occurs, but it is linked to being overweight (especially around the waist). South Asian people are more insulin resistant than Europeans, and this may be the reason why diabetes is much more

2

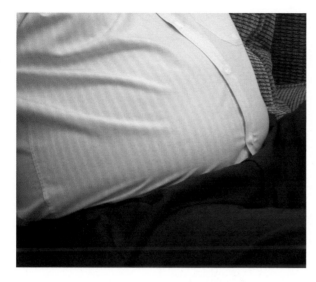

Figure 1.2
Central obesity
(excess weight
around the waist)
contributes to
insulin resistance.

common amongst South Asian people. We don't know why South Asian people are more insulin resistant, but it may be because our ancestors were able to survive with lower carbohydrate intakes. In the presence of plenty of carbohydrate, we develop diabetes.

- Insulin deficiency. There may be reduced levels of insulin released from the pancreas, due to the beta cells being destroyed (as in type 1 diabetes – see later) or the beta cells just cannot produce enough insulin to overcome the insulin resistance (as in type 2 diabetes).

As a result of these two problems, the glucose that is eaten in food is digested and absorbed normally, but does not enter the muscle, liver and fat cells, thus tending to stay in the bloodstream. Over time, high levels of glucose in the blood tend to have a damaging effect on various parts of the body.

What does not cause diabetes?

Diabetes is not contagious! Living with, or knowing someone with diabetes does not increase your risk of diabetes.

4

2 HOW IS DIABETES DIAGNOSED?

Who is at risk of diabetes?

In the UK there are 2.2 million people with known diabetes. It has been suggested that there is a 'missing million' – around 1 million people who suffer from diabetes but do not know about it. There are many people who have diabetes but do not realise it, as they have no symptoms at all. Diabetes may be picked up on a routine blood test, or perhaps following a medical check for employment or insurance purposes. At the moment, there is no formal screening programme for diabetes, but it is worthwhile getting your blood checked by your GP regularly, if you are at high risk of diabetes, people such as:

- those of South Asian or Afro-Caribbean descent
- those over age 50 years
- those with a strong family history of diabetes, for example, in your mother, father, brothers or sisters
- those with a previous diabetes during pregnancy
- those who are overweight (high body mass index or waist circumference).

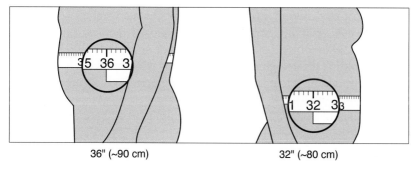

36" (~90 cm)   32" (~80 cm)

Figure 2.1   Increased waist circumference increases risk of diabetes.

The **body mass index** (BMI) is worked out by dividing your weight (in kilograms) by your height (in metres) squared, that is, multiplied by itself. A normal BMI in South Asian people is between 18 and 23. A value of between 23 and 28 is classed as overweight, and over 28 is classed as obese. Waist circumference above 90 cm (36 inches) in South Asian men and 80 cm (32 inches) in South Asian women confers a greater risk of diabetes.

What are the symptoms of diabetes?

As stated above, some people do not develop symptoms. However, if your blood glucose sugar is quite high, you may get the following symptoms:

- thirst and drinking water very frequently
- passing a lot of urine, especially at night
- rapid weight loss – loss of over 5% of your body weight over a short period of time is very significant
- severe tiredness
- frequent skin infections – abscesses and boils occurring frequently should alert you to having a glucose check
- excessive hunger
- blurred vision.

What tests are required?

If you have symptoms such as those above, your GP or nurse will probably check a **capillary blood glucose**. This involves a fingerprick test of your blood, using a meter to test the glucose level in the blood. If you have fasted, a capillary blood glucose over 7.0 is significant. If you have eaten, a capillary blood glucose above 11.1 is also significant. Please note, however, that you should not be diagnosed diabetic only on the basis of a capillary blood glucose. Your doctor or nurse should also send you for a **fasting plasma glucose** test, which is done by taking blood from a vein, and sending it to a laboratory. Blood glucose is measured in millimoles per litre (mmol/l) in the UK.

The results of your fasting glucose tests will come back with one of three results:

- normal: less than 6.0 mmol/l. This means it is unlikely you have diabetes;

- impaired fasting glucose (IFG): between 6.1 and 6.9 mmol/l. If your fasting glucose comes back at this level, your GP or nurse should book you for an oral glucose tolerance test (see below);
- diabetes: 7.0 mmol/l or above. If you have no symptoms, ideally a fasting glucose should be done twice to confirm you have diabetes.

Oral glucose tolerance test (OGTT)

This test is performed if your fasting glucose test is in the IFG range. The test is usually done in a hospital outpatients department or diabetes centre, although some GP practices may also do the test. To prepare for the test, you will need to fast from midnight the night before. You can drink water, but you must avoid food and any other drinks. The test is usually done at 9.00 a.m., when a fasting blood test will be done, and you will be asked to drink a solution with 75 g of glucose. Many centres use the equivalent glucose dose in a glass of Lucozade, which is much easier to drink. A further blood test will be taken 2 hours later.

The results will come back showing four possibilities as shown in Table 2.1.

Table 2.1   Results of the OGTT for diabetes

Fasting glucose	2-hour glucose	Classification
Less than 6.0	Less than 7.8	Normal
6.1–6.9	Less than 7.8	Impaired fasting glucose
Less than 7.0	7.8–11.0	Impaired glucose tolerance
7.0 or above	11.1 or above	Diabetes

What does impaired fasting glucose (IFG) mean?

If you have been told you have impaired fasting glucose, this means that you are at risk of developing diabetes in the future. You should have an OGTT to ensure you are not diabetic. If this is normal, you will probably need a fasting glucose test yearly. You can reduce your risk of diabetes by improving lifestyle and losing weight (see later).

What does impaired glucose tolerance (IGT) mean?

Impaired glucose tolerance indicates that after food, your glucose goes higher than it should do. This is probably due to insulin resistance. IGT is a high-risk state for developing diabetes and is also called **pre-diabetes**. If left untreated, around 10% of people will become diabetic each year. If you have IGT, you should make a determined effort to lose weight, as a 5% weight loss can lead to a 50% reduction in the risk for developing diabetes in the future (see later).

3 HOW COMMON IS DIABETES?

Diabetes is common, and becoming more common worldwide. There is currently an epidemic of diabetes, with numbers of people diagnosed with the condition rising year on year. It is estimated that there are 171 million people worldwide with the condition, but by 2030, this will rise to 336 million. In the UK, it is known that 2.2 million people have the condition, and a further 1 million have the condition, but do not know about it. By 2010, estimates are that there will be 3 million people with diabetes in the UK.

With regard to South Asian people, it has been estimated by the World Health Organization that by the year 2030, around one-third of all patients with diabetes will reside in the Indian subcontinent. The risk of type 2 diabetes (see later) in South Asians is about four to five times as high as that in Europeans, and around 1 in 4 South Asian adults over the age of 50 have diabetes. Over a lifetime, a South Asian person has about a 1 in 3 chance of developing diabetes. The condition also tends to develop earlier (by around 10 years), and complications of diabetes, such as kidney disease and heart disease, develop much more frequently compared to Europeans.

If you have recently been diagnosed with diabetes, don't worry – you are not alone!

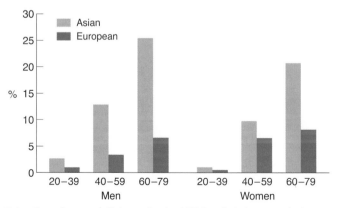

Figure 3.1   Prevalence of diabetes in the UK South Asian population.

4 TYPES OF DIABETES

What is type 1 diabetes?

Type 1 diabetes used to be called **insulin-dependent diabetes**. In type 1 diabetes, the pancreas is unable to produce insulin. This is because the pancreatic beta cells have been destroyed due a phenomenon called **autoimmunity**. This means that the body attacks itself, because it recognises the beta cells as foreign, and hence destroys them. We do not know why this happens, but there appears to be a strong inherited component. Other explanations may be that there is infection with a specific virus or bacteria, there has been exposure to food-borne chemical toxins, or there has been exposure as a very young infant to cows' milk, where an as yet unidentified component triggers the autoimmune reaction. A person who has a brother or sister with type 1 diabetes has about a 1 in 6 chance of developing type 1 diabetes themselves. Type 1 diabetes usually starts in childhood or young adulthood, although it may be seen in older people. People with type 1 diabetes must have injections of insulin to survive. The condition tends to be more common amongst North European people, especially in Scandinavia, although there are pockets of high numbers with the condition in other areas.

What is type 2 diabetes?

Type 2 diabetes used to be known as **maturity-onset diabetes** or **non-insulin-dependent diabetes** (NIDDM). In type 2 diabetes, there is insulin resistance (insulin does not work as well as it should to reduce blood glucose), with varying levels of insulin deficiency. This type of diabetes tends to affect older people, although we are now seeing rising rates of type 2 diabetes in children and young adults, due to the increasing problem of obesity. Increased risk of type 2 diabetes is conferred by:

- increasing age
- being overweight and obese

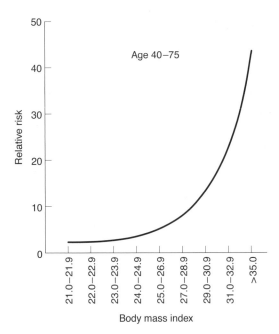

Figure 4.1 The risk of diabetes is very much increased by increasing BMI.

- physical inactivity
- being South Asian or Afro-Caribbean.

Some differences between type 1 diabetes and type 2 diabetes are shown in Table 4.1.

Table 4.1 Differences between type 1 and type 2 diabetes

Type 1	Type 2
Sudden onset of symptoms	May have no symptoms, or come on very slowly
Tends to be younger people	Tends to be older people
More common in northern European people	More common in South Asian and Afro-Caribbean people
Family history of diabetes in around 10%	Family history of diabetes in around 30%
Needs insulin to survive	Can be treated with lifestyle change, tablets or insulin
Patients are usually slim	Patients are often overweight

Other causes of diabetes

Less common causes of diabetes include:

- medication, such as steroids (used for inflammatory conditions, such as asthma, arthritis), tablets for psychiatric problems, blood pressure tablets (beta-blockers and thiazides);
- pregnancy: gestational diabetes occurs in pregnancy, and can have adverse effects on the health of the baby. It usually goes away after delivery;
- pancreatic disease: chronic pancreatitis and cystic fibrosis damage the pancreas, leading to insulin deficiency;
- hormonal problems: diseases of the thyroid and adrenals can also lead to diabetes, although this is very uncommon.

5 WHAT ARE THE COMPLICATIONS OF DIABETES?

Diabetes can have very serious effects on health, and complications of diabetes can arise 5–10 years after diabetes is diagnosed. As many people may have type 2 diabetes for a number of years before they are diagnosed, they may already have developed complications by the time they are diagnosed.

This section explains some of the potential problems that can occur if diabetes is poorly managed. Whilst these complications can be very serious, it is important to remember that with good management, the risk of developing complications is very low.

The complications of diabetes can be divided into **acute** (sudden) and **chronic** (long-term).

Acute complications of diabetes

These can be due to very high glucose levels (**hyperglycaemia**) or very low glucose levels (**hypoglycaemia**).

Hyperglycaemia

In most people, high blood glucose levels (14 or above) do not cause acute problems, so long as they improve over time. If blood glucose levels are very high, and remain high, they can lead to an acute hyperglycaemic emergency. In people with type 1 diabetes, this can lead to **diabetic ketoacidosis (DKA)**, where a lack of insulin leads to use of fat as a fuel for the cells, which leads to the production of **ketone bodies**. These ketone bodies are acidic, and can turn the blood acidic, leading to major problems with the way the body's organs can work. Ketones in the blood can be checked with a ketone meter, although it is more usual to test the urine for ketones. Without urgent treatment with intravenous insulin, fluid and careful management in hospital, this condition can become rapidly fatal.

In type 2 diabetes, the hyperglycaemic emergency is called **hyper-osmolar hyperglycaemic syndrome** (HHS – formerly called 'HONK'). This condition is characterised by very high levels of blood glucose (usually greater than 20), and severe dehydration, which can lead to kidney failure or stroke. It needs urgent treatment in hospital.

Symptoms of a hyperglycaemic emergency include acute symptoms of diabetes (thirst, passing lots of urine, weight loss, etc.), tiredness, confusion or coma. In DKA, the patient may be breathing very rapidly and deeply, and may have a sweet smell (like 'pear-drops') on the breath – these are ketones (sometimes called 'ketone bodies').

If you have diabetes, and are becoming unwell, with high blood sugars, severe symptoms, and ketones in your urine, you should obtain medical advice as soon as possible.

Hypoglycaemia

Hypoglycaemia (also called a **hypo**) is defined for practical purposes as a blood glucose level of less than 4 mmol/l (many people say 'four's the floor'), although many people have very few symptoms until glucose levels are around 3.6 mmol/l. In humans, blood glucose is regulated very carefully between 4 and 7 mmol/l, by regulatory hormones, which include insulin. If the blood glucose drops, a number of **counter-regulatory** hormones kick in, which try to raise your blood glucose.

Diabetes itself does not cause hypoglycaemia, but hypoglycaemia occurs in people with diabetes, usually due to treatment with tablets or insulin. There may be a variety of reasons for why hypos occur:

- missed or delayed food
- too much insulin or diabetes medication
- vigorous physical activity
- drinking alcohol.

Hypoglycaemia can be dangerous if not picked up early. Fortunately, most people get very good warning signs, and are able to treat a hypo rapidly and effectively. Symptoms of hypoglycaemia include:

- hunger
- shakiness
- sweating

- anxiety
- weakness or dizziness.

If the hypo is not treated at this stage, more severe symptoms can occur;

- bizarre or aggressive behaviour
- confusion or appearing 'drunk'
- fits
- coma.

Sweating at night or waking up with headaches may be due to nocturnal (night-time) hypoglycaemia. In this circumstance, checking blood glucose levels at night, or having a 24-hour continuous glucose monitor (CGM) may be useful.

Hypoglycaemia can have a damaging effect on health. Prolonged hypoglycaemia leading to coma may lead to fatal brain damage. Hypos whilst driving, swimming or working at heights can lead to severe consequences. Very frequent hypoglycaemia has been suggested as contributing to memory loss. Some people who suffer from frequent hypos may develop **hypoglycaemia unawareness**, in which they are unable to get warning signs of a hypo, and end up collapsing. This can of course be extremely dangerous, especially whilst driving a car. If this is happening to you, you must consult a specialist in diabetes for advice on how to manage this problem, and you must immediately stop driving. If a hypo occurs whilst you are driving, you should stop your vehicle as soon and as safely as possible, remove the ignition key and move to the passenger seat, and treat as below. Only restart driving when your glucose levels have recovered to normal.

Treatment of hypoglycaemia is usually straightforward, and requires about 15 g of glucose using the following foods:

- half a glass of fruit juice or non-diet fizzy drink
- 2–3 glucose tablets
- 5 fruit pastilles.

You should be careful to avoid over-treating. After having some glucose, it is a good idea to have some starchy food with a lower glycaemic index (for example a sandwich), to stabilise glucose levels.

If you are too confused to eat or drink, you can be given **Glucogel** in your mouth, at the side of the cheek. It should not be used in people who are unconscious. Loss of consciousness can be treated with **glucagon** injections given into the muscle, either by a paramedic, or by a trained member of your family. In hospital, intravenous glucose may be given.

Hypoglycaemia is an unfortunate side-effect of trying to achieve good blood sugars. If you are having hypos very frequently, you may need your therapy adjusted, and you should consult your diabetes specialist for advice.

Chronic complications of diabetes

The chronic complications of diabetes can be divided into **microvascular** (small blood vessels) and **macrovascular** (large blood vessels). Microvascular complications of diabetes include effects on the eyes, kidneys and nerves. Macrovascular complications include heart problems, stroke and circulatory problems in the legs.

How does diabetes affect the eyes?

Poorly controlled diabetes can cause problematic visual blurring in both eyes, due to high glucose concentrations causing changes in the curvature of the lens of the eye. Once glucose concentrations settle, the blurring usually disappears.

Diabetes is the main cause of blindness in people of working age. It is particularly important because it is a potentially preventable cause of blindness. Diabetes affects the small blood vessels at the back of the eye, or **retina** (thus the term **diabetic retinopathy**). Importantly, eye problems in diabetes may not be noticed by the patient, until the vision is significantly impaired, by which time it may be too late to do anything to help. It is therefore imperative that everyone with diabetes has a **retinal screen**. This is usually done using digital photography, after putting in eye drops to open up the pupil in order to get a good view. If you have diabetes, you must discuss with your health care professional how to get your eyes screened. Every area should have a **retinopathy screening programme**, sometimes in conjunction with local opticians. Using this system, early signs of retinopathy can be very easily detected, and treatment can be instituted to reduce the risk of the eye problem worsening. If you have significant retinopathy, you will be referred to a specialist eye clinic, where you may undergo laser therapy to the eyes (**laser photocoagulation**), which is sight preserving.

18

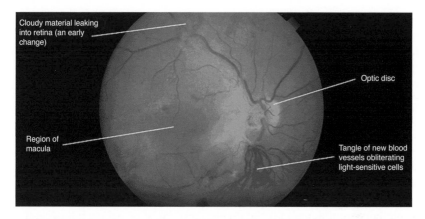

Cloudy material leaking into retina (an early change)

Optic disc

Region of macula

Tangle of new blood vessels obliterating light-sensitive cells

Figure 5.1 Diabetes can affect the retina leading to blindness.

People with diabetes are more prone to **cataracts**. The lens of your eyes is clear, and cataracts are areas of cloudiness or dark areas within the lens of your eyes, which may reduce your vision. If you have significant cataracts, a small operation can be performed to remove the cataract and

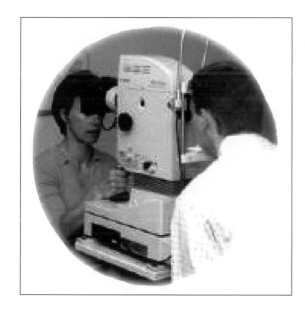

Figure 5.2 Regular eye checks can save your sight.

insert a replacement lens into the eye. It is also important to attend the opticians regularly to have a sight check and pressure check, because people with diabetes are also more prone to developing high pressure in the eyes – so-called **glaucoma**.

How does diabetes affect the kidneys?

The kidneys are two organs situated in your lower back, which have the role of filtering the blood. If the kidneys fail, impurities build up in the blood, leading to severe illness, and without treatment, can ultimately lead to death.

Diabetes can have a serious impact on the function of the kidneys (**diabetic nephropathy**), and is the commonest cause of kidney failure in the UK. High blood glucose, in combination with high blood pressure, leads to problems with the kidneys. The earliest sign of kidney damage is the presence of **protein** in the urine. This can be detected on testing the urine

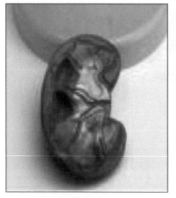 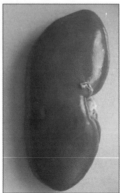 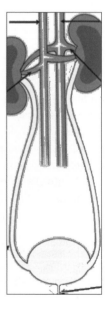

Figure 5.3   The kidneys filter the blood.

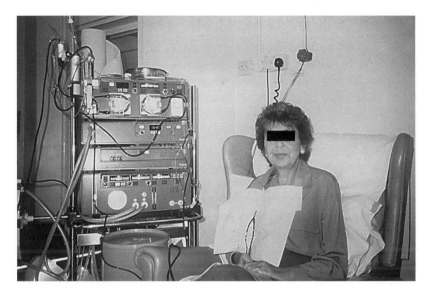

Figure 5.4 A patient having renal dialysis.

with special dipsticks, or sending the urine to the laboratory for testing. If there is protein in the urine, it is very important to improve blood glucose control, but also to improve blood pressure – aiming for a blood pressure under 125/75 mmHg (millimetres of mercury, see below for more information), if possible. The main treatment to reduce protein in the urine and prevent kidney failure, is to give **angiotensin converting enzyme** (ACE) inhibitors. These tablets appear to be protective for the kidney, reducing progression to kidney failure, but often a number of different blood pressure treatments are required to reduce the blood pressure to target levels (see treatment section).

Whilst developing kidney failure is not good, we are fortunate to have a number of effective treatments available. Kidney dialysis can be performed by a machine to which the patient is attached for around 3 hours a day for 3 days per week. Peritoneal dialysis can be performed using a tube into the abdomen. If possible, you might be suitable for a kidney transplant.

How does diabetes affect the nerves?

The nerves of the hands and feet are supplied with blood via very small blood vessels. These blood vessels can be affected in diabetes, leading to problems with the nerves (**diabetic neuropathy**). The nerves of the feet are most prone to be affected. You might notice numbness of the feet (like 'walking on cotton wool'), pins and needles, burning or shooting pains. These can be particularly bad at night. If you have neuropathy, you are more prone to developing foot ulcers. It is thus very important that you have your feet checked at least once a year for signs of neuropathy, and if you have neuropathy, you may need some education from a **chiropodist** to tell you how to prevent ulcers from developing. It is very important to have good nail care, well fitted shoes (not too tight, not too loose) and for you to look at your feet daily to ensure there are no breaks in the skin or blisters. Painful neuropathy can be treated using simple pain killers such as paracetamol, or stronger ones if required. Stronger tablets for neuropathy are available if painkillers don't work and your diabetes health professional should be contacted for advice.

Diabetes can affect other nerves too. In the hands, people with diabetes are more prone to developing pressure on a nerve in the wrist, leading to

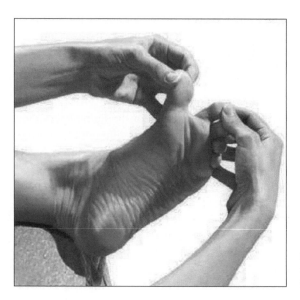

Figure 5.5 People with diabetes should check their feet daily.

burning, pins and needles and tingling in the fingers. This is called **carpal tunnel syndrome**, and can be treated with a small operation to release the nerve. Diabetes can affect the nerves that supply our blood vessels and other organs – this is called **autonomic neuropathy**. Autonomic neuropathy can cause many problems, such as dropping of blood pressure on standing up, frequent vomiting or diarrhoea, constipation, urinary problems such as incontinence or difficulty passing urine, or sweating with meals (**gustatory sweating**). These symptoms need specialist help – you should speak to your diabetes specialist if you are concerned.

Sexual problems

One problem that is common amongst diabetic men is **impotence**. This may be related to blood supply problems in the penis, or nerve problems due to autonomic neuropathy (see above), and can be very distressing for the patient and his partner. Around 50% of diabetic men over the age of 50 have difficulties with erections. Many men (especially South Asian men) find it difficult to discuss this problem with their health professional. It is important to discuss this issue, however, as there are very effective treatments available, in the form of tablets, injections and vacuum devices.

Diabetes and the heart

The most serious complication of diabetes is heart disease. Three out of every four people with diabetes will suffer heart disease. The most important heart problem is a **heart attack** (also called **myocardial infarction**). The heart is a pump made of muscle, supplied by large blood vessels. Build-up of **atheroma** or deposits within the heart blood vessels leads to blockage of the blood supply, and hence lack of oxygen to the heart muscle, and damage to the heart muscle. The most prominent feature of a heart attack is **chest pain**, which is often crushing, central, moving to the jaw or arms, accompanied by sweating and shortness of breath. An **angina attack** is similar, but usually less severe, and can be treated by using a spray of glyceryl trinitrate (GTN) under the tongue to open up the blood vessel. GTN does not usually help the pain of a heart attack. In some people with diabetes, there may be no chest pain with a heart attack. This is called a **silent myocardial infarction**. Urgent treatment is required in hospital with attempts to unblock the heart arteries with 'clot-busting drugs' or balloon

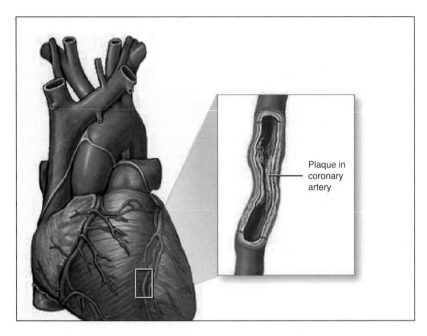

Figure 5.6   Insufficient blood flow to the heart muscle from narrowing of coronary artery may cause chest pain.

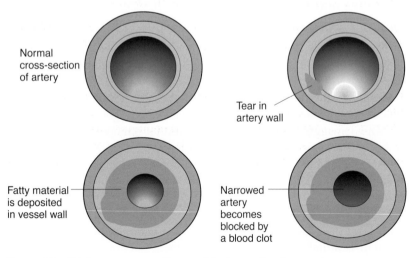

Normal cross-section of artery

Tear in artery wall

Fatty material is deposited in vessel wall

Narrowed artery becomes blocked by a blood clot

Figure 5.7   Diabetes can contribute to blockage of major arteries.

angioplasty (opening the artery with a balloon), and treatment to prevent complications, and recurrence of the heart attack.

Diabetes and stroke

People with diabetes are more likely than the general population to suffer from **stroke**. A stroke occurs when the blood supply to an area of the brain is interrupted, usually due to a clot in a brain artery, or less often due to a bleed from a brain artery. A stroke might present with a variety of symptoms, but most commonly it presents with weakness of one side of the body (arm or leg), weakness of the face, with facial drooping, and loss of or slurred speech. These symptoms may last for less than 24 hours, with full recovery – a so-called **transient ischaemic attack (TIA)**, or they may lead to a permanent weakness. Stroke is a major cause of death and disability, and is very often associated with uncontrolled blood pressure. There is no easy treatment for a stroke. 'Clot-busting drugs' such as those used in heart attacks are difficult to use in stroke, but may occasionally be used in the first 3 hours of the onset of a stroke. Treatment on a stroke unit, with intensive physiotherapy and rehabilitation, has been shown to improve outcomes in people who have had a stroke.

Diabetes and circulatory problems in the legs

Diabetic patients are more prone to developing **peripheral vascular disease (PVD)**. This is caused by clogging of the large blood vessels of the legs, and people with PVD often have symptoms of pain in the calves on walking a certain distance. This pain tends to feel like a cramp, and it becomes so severe that the person has to stop for a few minutes, and the pain settles. Poor circulation in the legs can also lead to problems with ulcers and gangrene, particularly if there is neuropathy as well. Treatment is aimed at increasing blood flow to the legs, and this can be achieved by balloon angioplasty (as in heart problems), or by a surgical bypass of the blockage.

6 TREATMENT TO PREVENT COMPLICATIONS

Complications of diabetes, whilst worrying, can be prevented. The key steps to prevention of complications are the following:

- education for people with diabetes and their families, to be empowered to self-manage their condition;
- monitoring of diabetes and regular screening for complications;
- improving the diet, increasing physical activity and stopping smoking;
- treating high blood glucose levels with lifestyle changes, tablets or insulin;
- treating high blood pressure;
- treating high blood cholesterol;
- thinning the blood with aspirin.

These areas will be covered in the next few chapters.

7 EDUCATION FOR DIABETES – WHERE CAN I FIND OUT MORE?

Whilst books like this are helpful for learning about diabetes, and will help you to manage your condition, it is extremely important to be given more information about diabetes and its effects on your body. You need to become an **expert patient** – having a clear knowledge about how to manage your diabetes. Most areas run education classes for diabetes, and whilst they may be time consuming, it is well worth the investment in time and effort to learn about your condition. In areas with large numbers of South Asian people, most units run South Asian language-based education sessions.

For people with type 2 diabetes, some educational packages have been recommended, although each area may have its own type of programme. Diabetes Education and Self Management for Ongoing and Newly Diagnosed (DESMOND) is widely used, as well as X-PERT. These programmes try to enable people to discuss their diabetes with other patients, and health professionals, and to develop a problem-solving approach. In type 1 diabetes, the equivalent programme is called Dose Adjustment for Normal Eating (DAFNE).

Why not find out what sort of diabetes education is offered in your area – ask your GP or nurse for advice.

8 HOW DO I MONITOR MY DIABETES?

Diabetes needs to be carefully monitored to ensure it is well controlled. You can undertake self-monitoring of blood glucose (SMBG) by a number of methods. Blood testing using a lancet and meter is commonly used (Figure 8.1). You can buy a meter from many pharmacists, but it may be a good idea to discuss which meter is the best with your diabetes health professional. Blood testing is particularly useful if you become unwell, or change therapy, or routine. If your diabetes is not well controlled, or you are on insulin therapy, you may need to test quite often. Remember, the test strips are very expensive, so if your diabetes is stable, you do not need to test very often – perhaps three times per week at different times (before breakfast and 2 hours after food) is adequate. Good pre-breakfast levels of glucose are between 4 and 7 mmol/l, and after food, up to 9 mmol/l, although some authorities would suggest lower levels. Some people prefer to check their urine for glucose. This has a place in well controlled diabetes treated with diet or tablets, so long as the tests are always negative, and you are having regular blood checks by your GP or nurse.

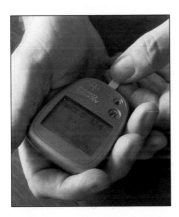 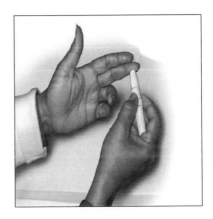

Figure 8.1   Self-monitoring of glucose levels is very important.

A very useful test that may be done to monitor diabetes is the **glycated haemoglobin** (also called glycosylated haemoglobin, or HbA_{1c}). This is a blood test taken from your vein, and gives a very useful measure of how good your blood sugar control has been over the previous 2–3 months. The higher the level of glycated haemoglobin, the poorer the blood glucose control. Levels of glycated haemoglobin that indicate good control vary according to the laboratory that does your test. Most laboratories suggest a level under 7.0% indicates good control, 7.0–8.5% as moderate control, 8.6–10.0% as poor control, and above 10% as very poor control. Ask your nurse or GP what your blood test shows, and what should be your target. This test should be checked at least twice a year.

Some people cannot have a glycated haemoglobin done because they have a slightly different haemoglobin type. In this circumstance, the laboratory may do a **serum fructosamine** test instead. This also gives an average for diabetes control over the previous 2–3 weeks. A level below 300 mmol/l suggests good control of diabetes.

9 WHAT SCREENING FOR COMPLICATIONS DO I NEED?

You must have regular screening for diabetic complications. Most people have this done by having a **diabetic annual review**. This should include the following:

- review of your health and how you are managing your diabetes;
- review of your medication;
- review of your glucose control, and whether you have had any problems with hypoglycaemia;
- advice and help on giving up smoking;
- check of your weight and BMI;
- check of your blood pressure;
- check of your urine for protein;
- check of your eyes for any sign of retinopathy. This should be done ideally using digital photography;

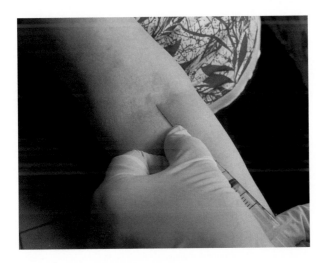

Figure 9.1
Blood tests should be done twice a year.

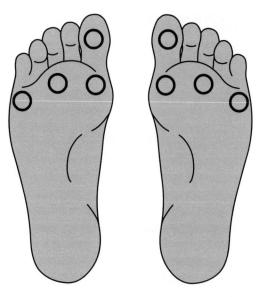

Figure 9.2 Feet should be checked for signs of neuropathy.

- check of your feet for signs of deformity, callus formation, ability to feel fine touch (using a special monofilament test) and check of your foot pulses;
- blood tests for creatinine (for kidneys), glycated haemoglobin, cholesterol levels and also liver blood tests;
- discussion and plan for targets for your diabetes over the next year.

10 I HAVE DIABETES – WHAT CAN I EAT?

There is no such thing as a 'diabetic diet'. **Healthy eating** is what all of us should do, including people who do not have diabetes. Many people with recently diagnosed type 2 diabetes can achieve good blood sugar control by diet alone. Around 80% of people with diabetes are overweight, and weight loss is recommended for many people with diabetes;

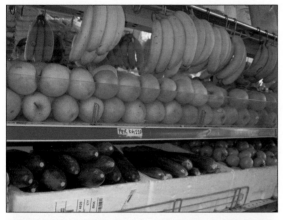

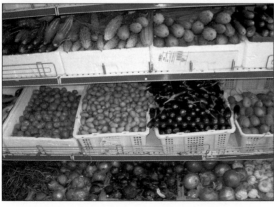

Figure 10.1 Fruit and vegetables are an important part of a healthy diet.

eating healthily will help achieve this aim. Learning about healthy food choices, and re-training your body to expect less food are the keys to managing your diabetes effectively.

People with diabetes should eat a diet which is:

- low in refined sugar
- low in saturated fat
- low in salt
- based around starchy carbohydrate foods such as pasta, bread, rice, chapatti, but portion sizes need to be controlled
- high in fruit and vegetable content (minimum of five portions daily).

Glycaemic index

Glycaemic index is worth knowing about. If you drink a glass of coca-cola, or eat a slice of white bread, the sugar enters your bloodstream very quickly; this means it has a **high glycaemic index**. This is useful if you are hypo, but not good if you have normal blood glucose, because the sudden rise in your blood glucose is difficult for your body to cope with. It is far more preferable to have a slow rise in blood glucose, by eating foods which release glucose into your bloodstream slowly – they have a **low glycaemic index**. High glycaemic index foods include fruit juice, non-diet fizzy drinks and white bread. Lower glycaemic index foods include basmati rice, pasta, yams, apples, whole grain seedy breads and low-fat yoghurt.

Should I eat 'diabetic foods'?

Many shops sell 'diabetic foods', but these are of little use, because they are high in fat, rather than sugar. Avoid them, and eat healthily!

Can I eat fruit?

Eating fruit is good for you. All fruits are suitable for you even if you have diabetes. Large portions of fruit (especially melons, mangoes, papaya and grapes) will elevate your blood glucose, but it is good to spread two or three small portions of fruit through the day. If you prefer tinned fruit, buy those in natural fruit juice, not syrup.

How do I reduce my fat intake?

Fatty foods have high calorific values, and will lead to you gaining weight. Animal fats, butter, ghee, cream and high-fat meat contain large quantities of cholesterol, which can contribute to arteries becoming clogged up. Try to avoid frying foods, and use other methods such as steaming, grilling or roasting. Low-fat and skimmed dairy products are preferable, and you should try to spend some time trimming off all visible fat from meat, and remove the skin from poultry. Prawns, eggs and avocados are fine to eat occasionally, but do not mix them in rich creamy sauces or dressings. Oily fish, such as mackerel, herring, salmon, sardines and fresh tuna are particularly good for your health.

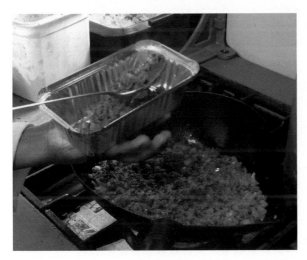

Figure 10.2 Cut down on fried food.

How do I lose weight?

Losing weight is one of the greatest challenges we can face. When high-fat foods are all around us, it is very difficult to resist. Nevertheless, losing weight is possible, and very desirable to help you control your diabetes. One pound of fat has around 3000 calories, and it is easy to pile this on, if we eat more calories than we burn. The secret is to eat less and do more!

Be realistic, and set achievable small goals within a set timeframe. An achievable goal, which would make a significant positive impact on your health is a 10% weight loss, which should be lost gradually (1–2 pounds per week – more rapid, and you are liable to regain what you lost). Reducing snacks, alcohol and second helpings are a good way to reduce your calorie intake. There are tablets that can help with weight loss as part of a healthy lifestyle. Discuss them with your diabetes health professional.

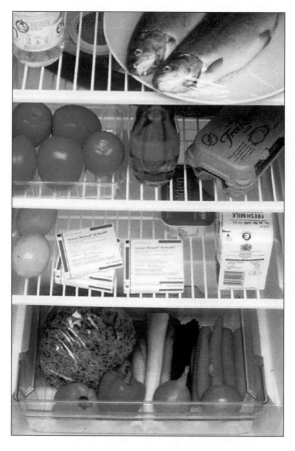

Figure 10.3   A healthy fridge of a patient treated with insulin.

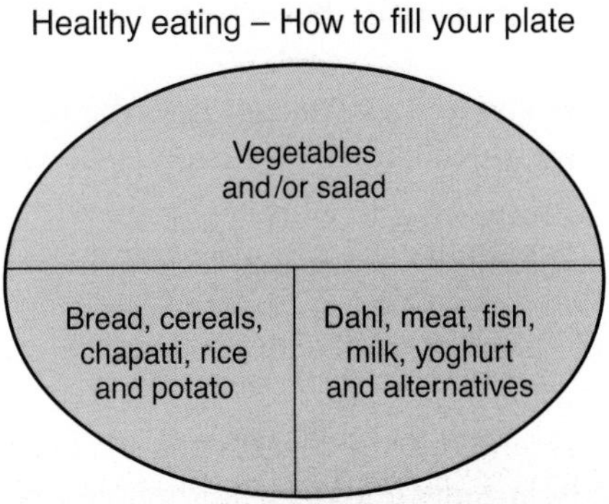

Healthy eating – How to fill your plate

Figure 10.4 Reduce your portion sizes. Look at the food on your plate.

Vegetables and/or salad

Bread, cereals, chapatti, rice and potato

Dahl, meat, fish, milk, yoghurt and alternatives

What about South Asian foods?

The following are some tips with South Asian foods:

- Rice is commonly over-eaten. Remember that **one plate of rice is equivalent to 18 cubes of sugar**. Try to cut down, and fill up on vegetables instead. Try to aim for less than half a plate of rice per day – it will make a big difference to your blood glucose levels. Basmati rice has a slightly lower glycaemic index compared to standard long grain rice.
- Make chapattis with little oil and ghee, and don't spread oil or ghee on them after cooking.
- Avoid adding butter when cooking rice.
- Try to avoid ghee and use less oil in cooking. If your food has a layer of oil floating on top, you are using far too much oil. Try different methods of cooking, for example grilling, roasting, tandoori, and use olive oil if possible. Try oil spray rather than pouring oil in your pan.
- Samosas and bhajias contain more saturated fat than fish and chips or burgers. It is also impossible to eat just one! Avoid them if you can.
- Measure the amount of oil you use – use a teaspoon rather than pouring straight into the pan.
- South Asian sweets are bad news for people with diabetes! They contain huge amounts of fat and sugar. Whilst these are sometimes difficult to avoid, try limiting to only one on special occasions. This is easier said than done, but reducing will make a big difference.
- Avoid sugar in hot drinks, and use calorie-free artificial sweeteners.

- Have only one glass of pure fruit juice per day – have the rest as whole fruit.
- Drink plenty of fresh water, 8–10 standard glasses per day. We often feel we are hungry when in fact we are thirsty, so start each meal with a glass of water.
- Avoid biscuits, but if you feel tempted, try dry biscuits such as Rich Tea, Morning Coffee or Ryvita with raisins.
- Increase your vegetable intake by having a salad with your main meal, and adding vegetables to meat curries.
- Dahl, chick peas, moong, peas and kidney beans are excellent sources of soluble fibre, which help reduce glucose and cholesterol levels. Try eating these more often.
- Cut down on red meat, and choose lean meat from the butchers. Chicken or turkey are healthier options, but remove the skin first.
- Try using a non-stick pan to reduce the amount of oil needed to cook.
- Eat oily fish more often (herring, mackerel, salmon, sardines, fresh tuna).
- Use semi-skimmed dairy products, low-fat yoghurt, low-fat evaporated milk and low-fat cheese.
- Reduce your salt intake, and use flavours instead – lemon juice, mixed spices, garlic, chilli and herbs. Be careful with pickles as they often are high in salt and sugar – use small amounts.

11 HOW MUCH EXERCISE SHOULD I DO?

Physical activity is very important in people with diabetes. Exercise can help to control your weight, blood glucose and blood pressure. Most authorities suggest 30 minutes of aerobic exercise each day is a good idea – this includes swimming, walking, jogging, cycling and dancing. If you have other medical problems (for example heart disease), you may need to seek medical advice before embarking on an exercise programme, but this does not mean that you should not exercise. Walking 2 miles a day three times per week can help reduce weight by 1 pound every 3 weeks, and regular uphill walking can help reduce weight by 14 pounds in only 3 months.

Walking is a particularly good exercise for people with diabetes. Walking helps improve your body's responsiveness to insulin, reduces weight, reduces cholesterol and blood pressure and reduces your risk of blood vessel complications related to diabetes. Thirty minutes of brisk walking each day is a very effective exercise. Why not buy a pedometer from a pharmacy, to help motivate you to build up your activity?

If you are treated with insulin, you do need to take more care before embarking on exercise. Check your blood glucose – if it is under 4.0 mmol/l, take a snack before exercising. Take care with exercise if your blood glucose is much above 14 mmol/l. Always carry some glucose tablets or a sweet drink to use if your sugar drops too low. If you plan on taking vigorous exercise, you may wish to cut your insulin dose slightly to counteract any hypoglycaemia you may encounter – seek advice from your diabetes health professional. If you have neuropathy or peripheral vascular disease (PVD), take care with exercises that cause pressure on your feet. Swimming might be a better option. Always wear socks and well fitting trainers.

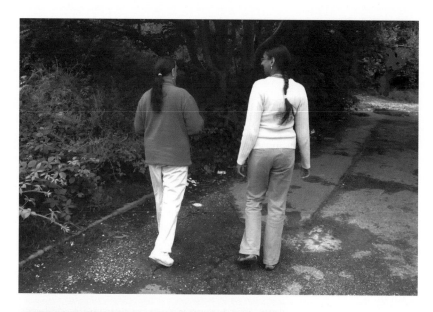

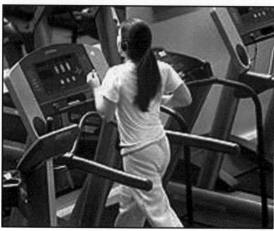

Figure 11.1 Exercise doesn't have to mean joining a gym – why not walk instead of driving?

12 WHY SHOULD I GIVE UP SMOKING?

Smoking and diabetes are bad bedfellows. Smoking can lead to the following:

- heart disease, stroke and circulatory disease
- premature death
- lung cancer
- chronic obstructive pulmonary disease
- poorer blood glucose control – smoking elevates glucose levels
- high blood pressure and cholesterol levels
- increased risk of blindness from retinopathy
- increased risk of kidney failure
- increased risk of impotence.

Stopping smoking can reduce your risk of a heart attack by up to 50%. It is not easy, but is absolutely essential for your long-term health. Many people succeed through a **smoking cessation programme** where you can get free tablets, nicotine patches or inhalators. Most areas run these – ask your GP or nurse. It also helps to join a group of people who are all trying to stop smoking.

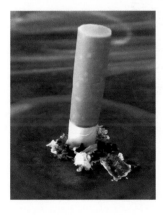

Figure 12.1   All people with diabetes MUST give up smoking.

13 WHY SHOULD I TAKE TABLETS TO CONTROL MY BLOOD GLUCOSE?

There is a lot of evidence that improved blood glucose control can reduce your risk of diabetes complications, especially the microvascular complications (see above). If you can maintain your glucose levels as suggested above, and your glycated haemoglobin below 7.0%, your risk for developing complications is low. If improving diet and exercise levels does not keep your diabetes under good control, your doctor or nurse may advise you to commence tablet treatment for diabetes. Tablets can be very effective in lowering your blood glucose, and work in a number of different ways. All treatments commonly used for diabetes have been subject to rigorous testing, and are extremely safe. Some tablets may have mild side-effects, but it is extremely important that you take your tablets regularly, as advised by your diabetes health professional. If you are worried by side-effects of the medication, discuss this with your diabetes health professional.

The tablet section (see Appendix) outlines the types of tablets available for treating blood glucose, their effects and side-effects.

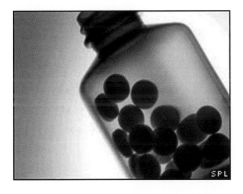

Figure 13.1 Tablets can control diabetes.

Should I try alternative therapies?

The tablets prescribed by your diabetes nurse or doctor have been rigorously tested, and found to be safe and effective. The same cannot be said for all alternative treatments. Whilst they may have a role for treating diabetes, many of the claims of the manufacturers of these drugs – in particular that they can 'cure' diabetes – are incorrect. If you plan to take alternative therapies, you MUST inform and discuss this with your diabetes health professional, and you MUST NOT stop your prescribed medication.

14   MY DOCTOR SUGGESTS I TAKE INSULIN. WHY IS THIS, AND HOW DO I TAKE IT?

Type 2 diabetes is a progressive condition. It frequently gets worse with time, despite efforts to improve your lifestyle and dietary habits. This is because the pancreatic beta cells become exhausted and are unable to produce insulin, even in response to the tablets.

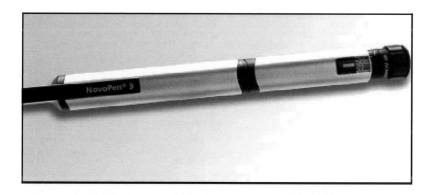

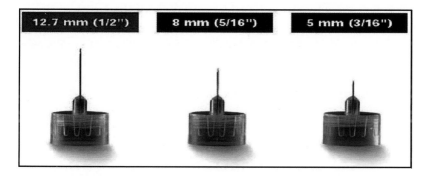

Figure 14.1   An insulin pen and needles.

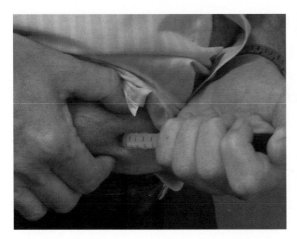

Figure 14.2 A person injecting insulin.

In this situation, your diabetes health professional might advise you to start insulin. Some reasons for starting insulin include:

- type 1 diabetes
- poor diabetes control despite good diet and lifestyle, and maximum doses of tablets (e.g. glycated haemoglobin above 7.5%)
- side-effects from, or problems with, taking tablets
- high blood glucose with severe symptoms
- pregnancy
- foot ulcers
- recent heart attack
- major surgery or illness.

Insulin cannot be given as a tablet, as it is rapidly broken down by the stomach and intestine. It is therefore necessary to give insulin as an injection. This sounds daunting, but it really is not difficult to give insulin. Most insulins are now available in pen devices, and are very simple to inject and use. Your health professional will teach you how to give the injections, and provide you with support and advice.

Insulin can be given in a number of ways (regimens).

Once-daily long-acting with tablets

In people with type 2 diabetes, once-daily insulin in addition to tablets can be used, with a long-acting insulin such as Insulatard, Humulin I,

Lantus or Levemir. This helps stop the liver releasing glucose overnight. It is useful for helping improve blood sugar control in people who do not have bad symptoms.

Twice-daily fixed mixture

Mixed insulin contains a percentage of short- and long-acting. For example, Novomix 30 contains 30% short-acting and 70% longer-acting insulin, whereas Humalog Mix 50 has 50% short- and 50% long-acting insulin. This can be given before breakfast and before an evening meal, and occasionally also with lunch. This regimen offers good blood sugar control, but you will have to have regular meal times and food intake.

Basal bolus

Short- or rapid-acting insulin is given before meals, and long-acting insulin is usually given before bed. This method offers the most flexible way of giving insulin. You can vary your doses, meal times and food amounts, and it works well for people who work shifts or travel a lot. It is also easy to adjust if fasting. It is the most common method of insulin treatment in people with type 1 diabetes.

The table in the treatment section (see Appendix) describes some of the insulins available, and how they work.

Some common reasons people give for not starting insulin are:

- 'If I go on to insulin, it means my condition is very bad'. This is not true. Insulin is used to prevent you developing problems with your health. Going on to insulin does not imply your health is worse.
- 'I knew someone who went on to insulin and suffered a heart attack shortly afterwards'. This is a common misconception that insulin made things worse. In fact, it is likely that this person's poor glucose control contributed to their heart problems. Insulin therapy is proven to reduce complications, not cause them.
- 'I don't want to gain weight'. Insulin can cause mild weight gain. If you continue to be strict with your diet and do plenty of exercise, the weight gain is usually minimal.
- 'I am worried about going hypo'. Insulin can cause hypoglycaemia, but this is uncommon, usually very easily treated, and rarely a major

problem, especially in type 2 diabetes. It is far worse to have high blood glucose than the occasional low one.

- 'I will lose my driving licence'. This is not true. You will not be able to drive a heavy goods vehicle, but you will be able to drive a car, and maybe even a taxi, with no problems. You MUST inform the DVLA and your insurance companies that you have diabetes and are commencing insulin. You will usually be given a 3-year renewable licence. If you are a taxi driver, you must inform the public carriage office, who will look at your circumstances individually.

- 'I am afraid of needles'. Many people state they are afraid of needles, but the needles to inject insulin are extremely thin and short, and most people can barely feel the injections. If you are able to monitor your blood tests, then giving insulin should really be no problem at all.

- 'A friend of mine got very blurred vision with insulin'. This can occur in the early stages of insulin therapy, due to changes in your lens, as a result of blood glucose fluctuation. This is temporary, and will get better within a few weeks once your blood glucose levels stabilise.

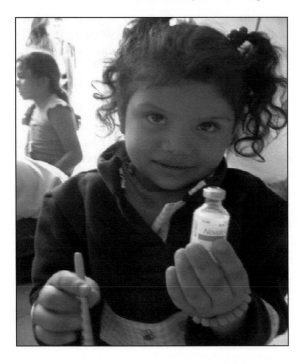

Figure 14.3 Even children with diabetes are able to give themselves insulin.

The following is some important information if you are being treated with insulin.

Injection sites

You must rotate your injection sites. Injecting into the stomach gives usually the most rapid absorption. If you are developing lumps or hard areas at your injection sites, you should avoid these areas.

Storage of insulin

You should store your insulin in the refrigerator until you come to use the insulin. Only take the pen or cartridge that you are going to start out of the fridge, and allow it to reach room temperature before using. Always ensure you have enough insulin to last you at least one week. Get a new supply before you run out.

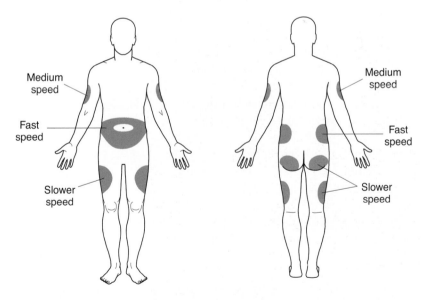

Figure 14.4   Injection sites.

Driving

Inform the DVLA and insurance company that you are taking insulin. Always check your blood glucose before driving, and do not drive if the glucose is under 4 mmol/l. Always carry around carbohydrate with you, and stop at least every 2 hours on long journeys, in order to eat and check your blood glucose.

Travel

Taking insulin when travelling abroad can be a challenge. Always carry a letter from your diabetes health professional stating that you have diabetes requiring insulin therapy. The insulin should be carried in your hand luggage (not in the luggage hold of an aeroplane, as it is likely to freeze). Test your blood glucose frequently. There is a simple rule of 'westwards, increase; eastwards, decrease'. If you are travelling to the Indian subcontinent, your day will be shortened, so you may need to reduce you insulin dose, or skip a dose, whilst if you are travelling to North America, you may need some extra insulin to cover extra meals. Discuss this with your diabetes health professional. Carrying your insulin around in areas with poor access to refrigeration can be a problem; try a Frio bag (www.friouk.com).

Advice on what to pack when travelling
- Blood glucose meter with enough glucose test strips.
- Enough insulin, pens, lancets for the entire trip.
- Adequate supplies of other prescription medications.
- Rapid carbohydrate, such as glucose tablets, sweets and non-diet soft drinks.
- Complex carbohydrate sources such as breakfast bars, crackers or fruit.
- Diabetes identification card.
- Travel insurance papers.
- Cool bag for your insulin (www.friouk.com).

Sick days

If you are unwell, and unable to take food, you should NOT stop your insulin. You should drink plenty of fluids, and try taking sips of soup or fruit juices. If you are completely unable to eat or drink, you must phone a health professional for assistance; you may require admission to hospital.

Disposal of sharps

Sharps should not be disposed of in the domestic waste, but should be put into a sharps bin (Figure 14.5a), and collected for correct disposal. Most areas have their own system for disposing of sharps; discuss with your diabetes health professional.

Identification

It is a good idea to have some sort of identification which shows you are a person with diabetes treated with insulin (Figure 14.5b).

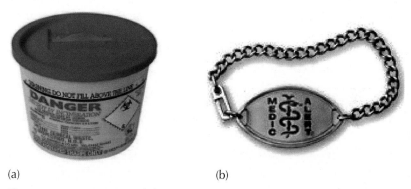

(a)   (b)

Figure 14.5   (a) Dispose of sharps in a sharps bin; (b) a Medic-Alert bracelet is a good idea.

15 WHAT IS HIGH BLOOD PRESSURE?

High blood pressure has been shown to increase the risk of complications of diabetes, including stroke, heart disease, kidney problems and eye problems. Treating high blood pressure if you have diabetes is extremely important. You should have your blood pressure checked at least twice a year, and if it is persistently high, you will need treatment. Blood pressure readings are given as two numbers, measured using millimetres of mercury (mmHg):

- systolic blood pressure: persistently above 140 mmHg in people with diabetes is too high;
- diastolic blood pressure: persistently above 80 mmHg in people with diabetes is too high.

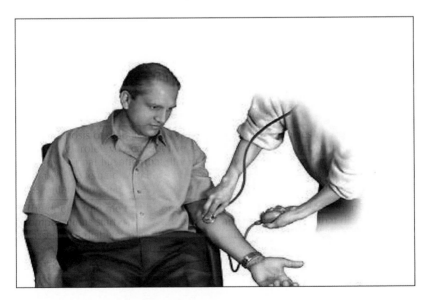

Figure 15.1   Every health care visit should include a blood pressure reading.

Thus, if your reading is regularly around 145/85 mmHg, this is too high, and should be treated.

How do I treat my high blood pressure?

Diet and exercise, with weight loss, may help. You should also concentrate on reducing your salt intake as this may also help to reduce your blood pressure. Your diabetes health care professional may advise you to start medication. This is very common; around 75% of people with diabetes need medication to treat their blood pressure. You may need two, three or four different medications to bring your blood pressure down. If your blood pressure is persistently above 140/80 mmHg, you should be started on medication, with an aim to bring the blood pressure down to below 130/80 mmHg, or under 125/75 mmHg if you have any protein in the urine. Some commonly used blood pressure tablets are listed in the treatments section (see Appendix).

16 WHAT IS A HIGH CHOLESTEROL?

Cholesterol is a type of fat in the blood. It is found in some foods, and some cholesterol in the diet is essential to keep us healthy. High levels of cholesterol, however, can be very harmful, as it can lead to deposits of **atheroma** on the arteries, leading to furring up of the arteries and blockage. This can lead to heart attack, stroke and circulatory problems. There are two types of cholesterol in our blood. Good cholesterol is called **high density lipoprotein (HDL)** cholesterol, and we benefit from having high levels of this. Bad cholesterol is called **low density lipoprotein (LDL)** cholesterol, and we benefit from having low levels of this. Another type of fat in the blood is called **triglycerides**. High levels of this may contribute to atheroma, but can also lead to inflammation of your pancreas, or pancreatitis.

You must have your cholesterol checked at least yearly. Your diabetes health professional may check just the **total cholesterol**, or a **full lipid profile**, which will include the LDL cholesterol, HDL cholesterol and triglycerides. If the latter is checked, it should ideally be done using a fasting sample.

Targets for lipid levels in people with diabetes are suggested as follows:

- total cholesterol less than 4.0 mmol/l;
- LDL cholesterol less than 2.0 mmol/l;
- HDL cholesterol above 1.2 mmol/l in women and 1.0 mmol/l in men;
- triglyceride less than 1.7 mmol/l.

How is cholesterol brought down?

Cholesterol comes from fatty, greasy, fried foods, and high-fat animal products (butter, ghee, cream, red meat, cakes, croissants, biscuits). Cutting out these animal fats, which are **saturated fats**, and using polyunsaturated fats such as olive oil or rapeseed oil, can bring your cholesterol down. Avoid using palm oil and coconut oil as they are high in saturated fats.

It has been proven that regularly eating oat-based cereals, especially porridge, fruit and vegetables, lowers your cholesterol. These foods have soluble fibre that binds fat from your food instead of allowing the fat to get absorbed into your bloodstream.

If your cholesterol is high, however, reducing it with tablets is the most effective way of improving things. These tablets, called **statins**, can reduce cholesterol by up to 50%. They have been proven to reduce heart disease and stroke in people with diabetes by around 30–40%. These drugs are so effective at reducing complications of diabetes, that recent guidelines have suggested that all people with diabetes over the age of 40 should be treated with statins, irrespective of their cholesterol levels. These tablets are very safe, and have very few side-effects (see Appendix).

17　WHY SHOULD I TAKE ASPIRIN?

Aspirin is a very old treatment, originally used for pain relief. It is now finding more uses, particularly in preventing blood vessel blockages. Aspirin is an **anti-platelet agent**. Platelets cause your blood to clot when you cut yourself. There is some evidence that platelets become too 'sticky' in people with diabetes. Aspirin can help reduce this 'stickiness', and reduce the risk of stroke, heart attack and circulatory problems. It is suggested that all people with diabetes over the age of 40 should be on aspirin provided their blood pressure (BP) is well controlled. You may wish to discuss this with your diabetes health professional.

18 OTHER ASPECTS OF LIFE WITH DIABETES

I have diabetes and want to have a baby. What should I do?

If you have diabetes, you must try to get very good blood glucose control BEFORE getting pregnant. This is because poor blood glucose control prior to pregnancy can lead to problems with the baby. You should be aiming for a glycated haemoglobin less than 7.0% before even trying to get pregnant. If you have type 2 diabetes treated with tablets, you should ideally be converted to insulin. You MUST take folic acid at a higher than normal dose of 5 mg daily (not 400 µg daily, which is normally suggested), to reduce the risk of your baby developing spina bifida. If you have diabetes and plan to get pregnant, you should discuss this carefully with your diabetes health professional.

Driving and life insurance

Remember to inform the DVLA and your insurance company that you have diabetes. You MUST inform them if you commence on insulin therapy. Life insurance can be more expensive if you have diabetes. Try specialist insurers through Diabetes UK.

Employment

There are very few jobs you can't do if you have diabetes. It is important to inform your employer of your new diagnosis, especially if you do go on to insulin. The need for regular meal breaks should be reiterated. If you start insulin, there may be some jobs you can't do (e.g. diving, roofing, HGV driving). Consult your employer or contact Diabetes UK for advice.

Fasting

Fasting can be very difficult if you have diabetes, especially during the long days. If you are treated with insulin, most Muslim authorities agree that you are exempt from fasting. If you decide to fast, you may need some changes in your tablets. You MUST seek advice from your diabetes health professional.

Some tips when fasting

- Do not stop taking your diabetic medication. Your doctor or nurse can advise how to alter your treatment during fasting, if this is necessary.
- You must take your medication according to what you have been advised. Timing of your medication may need to change; your doctor or nurse can advise you.
- At Suhur time (meal before dawn) try to eat your normal amount of food. If you do not feel like eating your normal food, eat a suitable alternative, but eat enough.
- If you feel unwell or get 'hypo' symptoms during the daytime, you should break your fast for that day.
- At Iftar time (meal after sunset) try not to eat sweet or fried food. Eat instead more fruits or lower fat snacks.
- Monitor your glucose control by doing blood tests. Blood tests can be done 2 hours after the Iftar meal and before the Suhur meal, but also at other times during the fast. Record your results in a diary.
- If your doctor has changed your medication for Ramadan, remember that at the end of Ramadan you should go back to your original dose of your diabetic medication.

19 I HAVE DIABETES. HOW CAN I PREVENT MY CHILDREN FROM DEVELOPING IT?

You are correct that your children are at risk of developing diabetes, because you have developed the condition. It is very important to try and educate your children to reduce their risk of diabetes.

There is now a great deal of evidence that diabetes is preventable in people who are at high risk. In people with impaired glucose tolerance (see above), who are at very high risk of developing diabetes, weight loss of 5% can lead to around a 50% reduction in risk for the development of diabetes.

The best way to prevent diabetes is to ensure that we lead a healthy lifestyle and do not gain weight as we get older. Regular exercise is a very important factor. A brisk walk of 30 minutes per day can help to reduce weight and reduce the risk of diabetes. Eating fruit and vegetables (at least five portions a day) regularly will also help. Reducing very sugary foods or fried/fatty foods is very important, not only to reduce the risk of diabetes, but also to reduce the risk of heart problems.

At the moment, there is no cure for diabetes once it develops. It is a condition that is chronic and lifelong, and the treatments available only control the problem, not cure it. There are some newer tablet treatments that may reduce the progression of diabetes. More recently, transplanting pancreas cells has shown some promise, but we are still far from a cure for this condition.

In the meantime 'stay healthy until a cure is found'.

20 SOME MYTHS AND MISCONCEPTIONS ABOUT DIABETES

This chapter deals with some myths and misconceptions about diabetes. These widely held myths are significant barriers to effective diabetes control.

Myths about diabetes	Facts about diabetes
Eating too much sugar causes diabetes. 'They say that there is a "sugar nerve" in the body that bursts.'	Not true. Being overweight and having a waist measurement of over 80 cm in a South Asian woman and 90 cm in a South Asian man makes you at risk of type 2 diabetes.
Diabetes is caused by a Western diet and stress, particularly family issues (getting children married and looking after elderly relatives, unemployment, overcrowding and fear of crime).	Not exactly. These do not cause diabetes, although they can be some of the trigger factors leading to the diagnosis of diabetes. For example, eating a lot of 'Western' fast foods and fizzy drinks can make you gain a lot of weight, making more demands on your insulin need. Stress releases 'stress hormones', which also make your body need extra insulin. If your pancreas can no longer make extra insulin, your blood glucose goes up and you develop diabetes.
More South Asian people suffer from diabetes than white British people – it's the 'shared blood' that causes it.	South Asian people have inherited the genes from their ancestors that make them more vulnerable to developing diabetes.
You cannot eat sugar or any sweet fruit or desserts when you have diabetes.	Not true. Table sugar, fruit, yoghurts and ice cream can be part of your total healthy diet, if eaten as part of your meals and in small portions.

Myths about diabetes	Facts about diabetes
You can catch diabetes. It is caused by something that gets into your body like a germ or some other bad thing from outside.	No, you develop diabetes because your own body can no longer meet the demand in the amount of insulin it needs. If a person in your family has diabetes, you have a greater risk of developing it.
You may only have a mild form of diabetes, not the severe one which needs insulin. Diabetes is really serious if you need insulin.	No, you either have diabetes or you do not. It is always a serious condition that needs to be treated and looked after well.
You can be cured of diabetes.	At present, there is no cure available. It can be managed with different treatments, which will need to be changed as the condition progresses.
People with diabetes must not exercise. Your body is weak. Exercise can make the illness or physical weakness worse. Ritual Muslim prayers (namaz) are a health-giving exercise.	This is a misunderstanding: physical activity is important in helping to control blood glucose levels. Namaz alone is not enough physical activity each day.
The diet for diabetes is very strict and you have to eat special foods, different from the rest of the family.	You should eat the same healthy diet advised for everyone. Special 'diabetic foods' are unnecessary, expensive and have no benefits for a person with diabetes.
There are herbs and alternative, traditional South Asian remedies, which can replace tablets or insulin.	Some herbal remedies may help lower blood glucose, but will not be enough on their own to treat your diabetes. At no time should you stop taking your tablets or insulin without first talking to your doctor or diabetes nurse.
Diabetes goes away when you go to Bangladesh or Pakistan. That shows diabetes is caused by the British weather (too cool) and lack of sun.	No, your blood glucose levels may go down in Bangladesh or Pakistan – because you are doing so much more physical activity there: you walk instead of using a bus or a train; you physically carry out many jobs that gadgets do for you in the UK (washing machine, electrical cooker and oven, water from tap).

Myths about diabetes	Facts about diabetes
Physical labour that makes you sweat is good for your health. In Britain, you don't sweat so much. That's why diabetes develops.	Diabetes is not linked to sweating a lot or a little. It is an imbalance in the amount of blood glucose and blood insulin that leads to diabetes. Physical activity is very important to help control diabetes.
You cannot drive if you have diabetes.	Not true. There are certain large vehicles – buses, trains, lorries and aeroplanes – which you will not be allowed to drive. You can drive a car or a van but you need to tell the DVLA and car insurance company if you need to start tablets or insulin.
You will not be able to get a job once you are diagnosed with diabetes.	There are some jobs that you will be unable to do: pilot, train driver, bus driver, fireman, ambulance driver, or deep sea diver. Diabetes should not stop you from getting work – the Disability Discrimination Commission is there to defend and assist you if you find barriers to employment.
You need to eat more if you feel weak and tired when you have diabetes.	Not entirely correct – you often feel weak and exhausted when your blood glucose is very high. You need either tablets or insulin – not more food – to help you regain your energy and strength.
I do not need to take my medicines when I feel well and I do not have any symptoms.	You need to continue to take your tablets and insulin – otherwise you will feel exhausted and ill again as your blood glucose gets higher.
Karela (bitter melon) can cure my diabetes. I know someone whose diabetes is treated with okra or grapefruit.	These do not cure diabetes. Karela, bilberries, or okra may help lower your blood glucose but you need to continue to take your medications or insulin.
I will develop diabetes complications no matter what I do. It is God's will. He has given it to me.	This is fortunately not true! You can avoid complications if you keep your blood glucose, cholesterol and pressure as low as possible. It is your responsibility to look after yourself.

67

Myths about diabetes	Facts about diabetes
Insulin will make me blind or cause a heart attack. That's what happened to my uncle and my neighbour.	No, starting insulin early in your diabetes journey can prevent any of these diabetes complications from happening. Those people did not develop the problems because they started on insulin – they might not have developed them if they had started on insulin much earlier.
I will be fine as long as I take the medications my doctor tells me to.	It is necessary to take the medications but that is not all: changes are needed to make your food choices healthier and control the amount you eat; you may need to lose some weight – from your waistline especially and become as physically active as you can.
People with diabetes should take vitamin supplements.	Not necessarily. You need to eat a varied, balanced selection of foods, especially fruit and vegetables, which will give your body all the necessary nutrients and vitamins. Your doctor or nurse will advise you if you at any time need some supplements, like iron in anaemia or folic acid in pregnancy.
First the doctor put me on a diet – that did not work. Then he gave me one tablet, then two, then three – now they don't work. Now he wants to start me on insulin – how do I know that the insulin will work?	Diabetes is a progressive condition and your doctor has to match the treatment to the stage of your diabetes where you are at any time. Sticking to a healthy diet with controlled portions will always be part of your diabetes treatment. Different tablets work in different ways to help lower your blood glucose, and your doctor needs to change them as and when he sees the tablet is no longer doing its job effectively. Ultimately, people with type 2 diabetes will need to take insulin as their body no longer makes enough of it.

Myths about diabetes	Facts about diabetes
Sport and organised physical exercise are inappropriate for women and older men. Sports clothing and footwear are 'not appropriate for South Asian people'. 'Our clothing and shoe-wear restricts South Asians and in particular South Asian women in participating in exercise on prescription. Swimming is an obvious example, but we are reluctant to wear tracksuits too.' 'I ask my nurse where I can go for exercise class or swimming but I don't get any answers.'	Non-sporting activities, physical movement need to be fitted into daily activities. Walking to work, parking farthest away from shops, gardening, house cleaning, family outings are a natural way of fitting exercise into one's daily routine. It is not necessary to wait for 'exercise on prescription' – every one of us has a pair of legs we can use.
Fast walking is inappropriate, especially for women, the elderly and those of high social status.	Walking is one of the best forms of physical activity and easily fitted into everyday activities.
'Big is beautiful' – large belly is a sign of wisdom and wealth.	No, central obesity is a sure sign of health risks, in particular, in people of South Asian and African origin. Fat stored in the front often leads to insulin resistance, diabetes and heart attacks.
It is OK to skip tablets to reduce unpleasant side-effects, especially if you are not eating traditional foodstuffs like roti, which have 'strengthening' properties and balance out the side-effects.	No, if you get unpleasant side-effects that you have not been warned about initially, it is important to contact your doctor or nurse. There is often an alternative that can suit you better.
Taking so many tablets over long periods is not good to your health. 'I don't want to die by taking so many. Taking so many medications together could counteract their individual effects. Instead of giving too many tablets why don't they give one instead?'	You need to take all the tablets as your doctor has prescribed; they work in different ways and some are for blood glucose, others for blood pressure, and others for cholesterol.
You only need to take all the tablets when your readings are high.	The tablets will help to lower the glucose readings – otherwise they go up again.

Myths about diabetes	Facts about diabetes
I stopped taking those tablets because they did not take away the pains in my feet. Another tablet did not improve my blood sugars at all.	Many tablets do not give instant relief of symptoms; the dosage often needs to be increased gradually (for example, gabapentin, amitriptyline), and it can take weeks to see their effect (glitazones).
It is difficult for us South Asians not to eat what is offered to us when you visit friends and relatives. You cannot refuse food that is offered to you, especially by an older relative. Refusal would cause offence.	It would be beneficial for you and your host(ess) to eat fruit, raw vegetables, or yoghurts as healthy snacks when entertaining. Biscuits, croissants and cakes have a lot of fat and sugar, which makes you put on weight.
'I get help and advice about my diabetes from my neighbour who has it too.'	The best source of diabetes information is your GP, diabetes nurse, or Diabetes UK (careline and leaflets available in most South Asian languages, too).
Some foods are hot, such as meat, fish, eggs, garlic, carrots, mangoes, dates, aubergine, lentils, coffee, tea, honey and mustard. Hot foods raise the body temperature, excite emotions and make you cheerful. In certain illnesses or pregnancy, you should avoid hot foods. Others are cool, like dairy foods, rice, wheat, potato, okra, coriander, cauliflower, ghee (butter), green leafy vegetables, most fruits and cucumber.	It is better to place foods into groups such as: protein, carbohydrate (starch) and fat. Based on this grouping, you can choose which foods to include in your meal and how much.
Control of diabetes requires restoring the body's internal balance by taking particular foods and fighting the 'germ' with medicine. The onset and control of diabetes depends on the balance of food entering the body and on balance exit of body fluids – semen, sweat, urine, menstrual blood, etc. Diabetes is a weakness in the body, caused by the internal stock running out.	Diabetes cannot be controlled by taking particular foods – it needs to be treated by tablets that help take the glucose from your blood to the body cells, tablets that help your body make more insulin, or both. When your body is no longer able to make enough insulin, it is vital to take insulin from outside your body – by either injecting or inhaling.

70

Myths about diabetes	Facts about diabetes
There are foods that are strong and others that are weak (depending on their nourishing power); 'digestible or 'indigestible' (digestibility). Strong foods give energy (white sugar, lamb, beef, ghee, solid fat and spices). They are good for the healthy body and for festive meals, but worsen those who are ill or old. Weak foods are preferred for every day meals and for the sick and old – foods such as boiled rice and cereals. Raw foods and grilled or baked foods are indigestible, as are all root vegetables. Elderly, ill and young people should not eat these foods.	This type of food classification does not apply to diabetes treatment. If you have diabetes, it is necessary to eat starchy foods in the right amounts (you can discuss this with your dietitian, diabetes specialist nurse, or practice nurse). Also you need to avoid eating too much fat as it leads you to gain weight and animal fat raises your blood cholesterol. This can cause a blockage in your blood vessels (heart attack, stroke, or a foot without proper blood supply). Eating fruit and vegetables every day, as well as oily fish at least three times a week, can prevent such problems from happening to you.
Baking and grilling alter the nature of the food, therefore are not suitable for South Asian cooking.	Baking and grilling are cooking methods that do not cause damage to parts of your body as you do not need to use fat when you grill or bake, instead of frying.
Chewing betel-quid ('paan') has positive health effects.	Chewing tobacco causes many types of cancer: in the mouth, stomach, food pipe, bowel and bladder. Paan chewing also damages your teeth and gums. It is extremely harmful to your health. You should get help and support to quit tobacco in any form.
The diagnosis of diabetes puts you into a 'sick role': you cannot live a healthy normal life after that. If you are a young female, you become less suitable for marriage.	Although diabetes is a serious lifelong condition, many people have proven that it is possible to live a healthy, active and full life, get married and have children.
'The doctor told me that before complications start, start wearing glasses. The diabetes may affect your eyes or your feet. So if you take the glasses, your eyes may be spared.'	Wearing glasses does not prevent any of the damage that diabetes can cause to your eyes. You can prevent such damage by attending your appointments to have your eyes photographed at least once a year at the retinal screening clinic.

Appendix 1   SOME COMMON TREATMENTS USED IN DIABETES

Treatments for high blood glucose

Tablet class	How does it work?	When is it used?	Possible side-effects
Biguanide: e.g. metformin	Reduces glucose output from the liver	Usually the first treatment for type 2 diabetes, especially if overweight	Can cause mild diarrhoea, and nausea. Reduced if you take with food, and usually settles with time
Sulphonylurea: e.g gliclazide, glimepiride, glibenclamide	Stimulates insulin release from the beta cell	May be second or third line after metformin	Hypoglycaemia if taken without food
Glitazones: e.g. rosiglitazone, pioglitazone	Improves sensitivity of the body to insulin	Second or third line after metformin. Occasionally used with insulin	Takes some months to work. May cause weight gain. Liver function tests need to be monitored. Some swelling of legs is seen occasionally. Can cause fluid accumulation on the lungs very occasionally – discuss with your doctor if you become breathless. Very recently, some studies suggest that rosiglitazone may cause increased problems with the heart. Data from large studies are awaited. If you are concerned, discuss the issue with your diabetes health professional

Tablet class	How does it work?	When is it used?	Possible side-effects
α-Glucosidase inhibitor: e.g. acarbose	Reduces absorption of glucose in the intestine	Third or fourth line after above, but many people get side-effects	Can cause diarrhoea and abdominal bloating
Meglitinides: e.g. repaglinide, nateglinide	Short-acting stimulators of insulin release from the pancreatic beta cells	Taken with meals – no meal, no tablet. May be helpful for erratic mealtimes/ fasting	Hypoglycaemia
Lipase inhibitor: e.g. orlistat	Reduces the amount of fat absorbed in the diet	Used as an aid to help weight loss in obese people	Fatty diarrhoea, abdominal pain, bloating
Appetite suppressant: e.g. sibutramine, rimonabant	Suppresses appetite	Used as an aid to help weight loss in obese people	Sibutramine can cause high blood pressure – should be avoided in hypertension. Rimonabant can cause nausea, anxiety and depression
DPP-4 inhibitor (Gliptin): E.g. sitagliptin, vildagliptin	Enhances production of insulin from the pancreas and reduces appetite	Third or fourth line after metformin	Nausea is sometimes a problem
Incretin mimetic: e.g. exenatide (Byetta)	Enhances production of insulin from the pancreas and reduces appetite. This is not actually a tablet. It is given by injection twice daily	Poor control on tablets, people with diabetes who are overweight. Studies have shown significant weight loss and improved glycaemic control	Nausea is a common a problem

Some common insulins

Type	Examples	How is it used?
Rapid-acting (analogue insulins)	Aspart (Novorapid), lispro (Humalog), glulisine (Apidra)	Rapid-acting insulin just before meals
Short-acting (human insulins)	Humulin S, Actrapid	Short-acting 20 minutes before meals
Intermediate-acting	Insulatard, Humulin I	Once daily usually at night either with tablets or with short-/rapid-acting insulin at mealtimes
Long-acting	Insulin glargine (Lantus), detemir (Levemir)	Once daily usually at night either with tablets or with short-/rapid-acting insulin at mealtimes
Mixed human insulins	Mixtard 30, Humulin M3	Taken 20 minutes before breakfast and 20 minutes before evening meal
Mixed analogue insulins	NovoMix 30, Humalog Mix 25, Humalog Mix 50	Taken just before breakfast and evening meal
Animal insulins	Hypurin Porcine Isophane, Hypurin Porcine Neutral, Hypurin Bovine Lente, Hypurin Bovine Neutral	Some people feel human and analogue insulins cause them problems with hypoglycaemia and prefer to use animal insulins. Use of these is rare nowadays

Tablets for blood pressure

Tablet class	How does it work?	When is it used?	Possible side-effects
ACE inhibitor: e.g. ramipril, lisinopril, perindopril, enalapril	Opens up blood vessels by reducing hormones that cause blood vessels to close	First line in most people with diabetes, especially if there is protein in the urine	Dry, tickly cough may occur. If this occurs, the tablet should be changed to another. Kidney blood test should be checked within two weeks of commencing this therapy
Calcium antagonist: e.g. amlodipine, felodipine, nifedipine LA	Opens up blood vessels by blocking calcium channels in the blood vessel wall	Second line to ACE inhibitors, although might be first line in Afro-Caribbean people	Swelling of the legs is common. Some people get flushing or headache
Thiazide diuretic: bendrofluazide, indapamide SR	Cause you to pass more urine, hence lower blood pressure	Second or third line	Low potassium levels may occur – this should be checked regularly. Impotence can occasionally occur
Beta-blocker: atenolol, bisoprolol	Reduces heart rate	Not often used in people with diabetes, unless you have had heart attack or have angina	Wheeziness, cold extremities, impotence
Angiotensin II blocker: irbesartan, losartan, valsartan, candesartan	Opens up blood vessels by blocking a hormone that causes blood vessels to close	These are often used in place of ACE inhibitors if you develop a cough	Kidney blood test should be checked within 2 weeks of commencing this treatment
Alpha-blocker: doxazosin	Opens up blood vessels by blocking receptors causing blood vessel closure	Fourth-line treatment	Can cause dizziness on standing

Tablets for cholesterol

Tablet class	How does it work?	When is it used?	Possible side-effects
Statin: pravastatin, atorvastatin, simvastatin	Blocks the production of LDL cholesterol	People with diabetes over the age of 40 years, or under 40 years with one other risk factor	Rarely liver inflammation can occur. Liver blood tests should be checked regularly. Some people develop mild muscle aches. If severe, treatment should be stopped
Fibrates: fenofibrate micro, bezafibrate (Bezalip Mono)	Helps reduce triglycerides, LDL cholesterol and elevate HDL cholesterol	People with high triglycerides (above 2.0 mmol/l)	Muscle aches can occur, especially when used in combination with a statin
Cholesterol absorption inhibitor: ezetimibe	Helps reduce absorption of cholesterol from the intestine	In combination with a statin if cholesterol levels remain high	None of note

Appendix 2   SOME USEFUL CONTACTS

- Diabetes UK Central Office
  Macleod House, 10 Parkway, London NW1 7AA
  Tel: 020 7424 1000
  Fax: 020 7424 1001
  E-mail: info@diabetes.org.uk
  Website: www.diabetes.org.uk
- The South Asian Health Foundation
  E-mail: info@sahf.org.uk
  Website: www.sahf.org.uk/index.html
- The American Diabetes Association
  Website: www.diabetes.org

Index